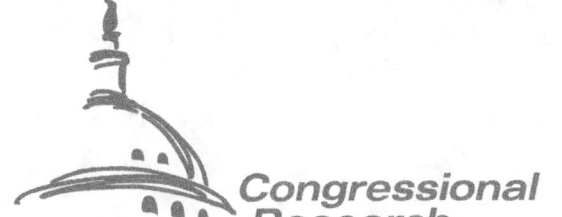

# Medigap: A Primer

**Carol Rapaport**
Analyst in Health Care Financing

September 19, 2012

Congressional Research Service
7-5700
www.crs.gov
R42745

**CRS Report for Congress**
*Prepared for Members and Committees of Congress*

# Summary

Medicare is a nationwide health insurance program for individuals aged 65 and over and certain disabled individuals. The basic Medicare benefit package (termed "Original Medicare" in this report) provides broad protection against the costs of many, primarily acute, health care services. However, Medicare beneficiaries may still have significant additional costs, including copayments, coinsurance, deductibles, and the full cost of services that are not covered by Medicare. In 2008, about 17% of Medicare beneficiaries purchased the private supplemental insurance known as Medigap to fill some of the cost gaps left by Original Medicare.

All Medigap plans cover some percentage of Medicare's cost-sharing. Some plans offer additions to these basics, including various combinations of greater coverage of Medicare cost-sharing, and care associated with foreign travel emergencies. The most popular plans are the most comprehensive, and cover all deductibles, copayments, and coinsurance not covered by Medicare. Medigap generally does not cover medical treatments not covered by Medicare, although it does extend coverage for certain covered services, such as coverage for additional hospital days beyond the Medicare benefit limit. Medigap is financed through beneficiary payments to the private insurance firms.

Federal law requires that Medigap insurers observe many consumer protections. Consumer protections are especially strong during open enrollment, which is a six-month period that begins for most individuals during the month they turn 65. During this period, individuals are protected against

- insurers refusing to sell them any Medigap policy that the insurer offers,
- insurers setting premiums based on the individual's health, and
- insurers imposing waiting times on the start of the policy, other than a maximum of a six-month waiting period for preexisting conditions.

Following the open-enrollment period, beneficiaries have other rights in limited situations, such as when they move to a different state. Guaranteed issue (or the right to buy a plan, to have the plan's premium not depend on health status, and in some cases to have the plan start coverage of preexisting conditions immediately) is one such right. The right of guaranteed renewability is available in a wide variety of situations, and genetic discrimination is forbidden. Moreover, Medigap insurers must pay out at least 65% (and sometimes 75%) of total premiums as claims to the beneficiaries.

Recent data show that Medigap premiums vary by states and other factors. A relatively small number of insurance firms sell Medigap plans. In addition, Medigap beneficiaries are concentrated in certain areas of the country and are more likely to have lower incomes than those holding employer-sponsored retiree health insurance.

The Patient Protection and Affordable Care Act (P.L. 111-148 as amended by P.L. 111-152, ACA) requests that the Secretary of Health and Human Services ask the National Association of Insurance Commissioners to review and revise existing standards to examine greater cost-sharing for Medigap beneficiaries. In addition, the President's 2013 budget proposal would provide incentives to increase cost-sharing. One rationale for these proposals is that beneficiaries on average reduce their use of medical care following an increase in cost-sharing. This decrease in medical care by Medicare beneficiaries could reduce Medicare expenditures and the federal deficit. On the other hand, if these reductions in medical care ultimately lower health status, the individuals might require more treatments or more expensive care.

This report provides a broad overview of Medigap insurance. The report covers the history of Medigap legislation, the various types of Medigap plans, consumer protections awarded to Medigap beneficiaries, and the requirements facing the insurance providers and the NAIC. Following an empirical description of Medigap markets, the report discusses proposals related to the percentages of a Medigap insurer's revenue that is returned as benefits to the policy holders and Medigap cost-sharing requirements.

# Contents

Introduction ........................................................................................................................................ 1
Medicare Coverage ............................................................................................................................ 2
Supplementing Medicare ................................................................................................................... 4
Medigap Plans .................................................................................................................................... 5
    History of Medigap Statutes ....................................................................................................... 6
        During the 1980s .................................................................................................................. 6
        During the 1990s .................................................................................................................. 7
        During the 2000s .................................................................................................................. 8
    Coordination of Payment Between Medicare and Medigap ....................................................... 9
    Plan Characteristics .................................................................................................................... 9
        Standardized Plans ............................................................................................................... 9
        Prestandardized Plans ......................................................................................................... 11
        Older Standardized Plans Available for Renewal Only ..................................................... 11
        Medigap Plans for States with Waivers ............................................................................. 11
        SELECT Plans ................................................................................................................... 12
        High-Deductible Plans ....................................................................................................... 12
    Plan Enrollment ........................................................................................................................ 12
Consumer Protections ...................................................................................................................... 14
    During the Open-Enrollment Period ........................................................................................ 14
    After the Open-Enrollment Period ........................................................................................... 15
        Guaranteed Issue ................................................................................................................ 15
        Guaranteed Renewal .......................................................................................................... 17
    Genetic Nondiscrimination ....................................................................................................... 17
    Switching Medigap Plans ......................................................................................................... 18
    Medigap for Individuals Under Age 65 ................................................................................... 18
Insurers' Requirements .................................................................................................................... 18
    Required Plans ......................................................................................................................... 19
    Premiums ................................................................................................................................. 19
    Medical Loss Ratios ................................................................................................................. 20
        Definition and Rationale .................................................................................................... 20
        Required Calculations ........................................................................................................ 20
The Role of the National Association of Insurance Commissioners ............................................... 21
Descriptions of Medigap Markets .................................................................................................... 22
    Medigap Premiums and Plan Choice ....................................................................................... 22
    Medigap Market Participation by Individuals Across States ................................................... 23
    Medigap Markets by Characteristics of Enrollees ................................................................... 24
Current Policy Issues ....................................................................................................................... 25
    Increasing Medical Loss Ratios ............................................................................................... 25
    Increasing Cost-Sharing ........................................................................................................... 26

# Figures

Figure 1. Sources of Supplemental Coverage Among Medicare Beneficiaries, 2008 ...................... 5

Figure 2. Distribution of Medigap Plans, All Medigap Beneficiaries, 2010 ................................. 13
Figure 3. Medigap Enrollment, by State, 2010 ........................................................................... 23
Figure 4. Percent of Medicare Enrollees with Medigap Coverage, by State, 2010 ...................... 24

## Tables

Table 1. Select Original Medicare Cost-Sharing Levels, 2012 ....................................................... 3
Table 2. Standard Medigap Plans, Effective On or After June 1, 2010 ........................................ 10

## Contacts

Author Contact Information ......................................................................................................... 27

# Introduction

*Medicare* is a nationwide health insurance program for individuals aged 65 and over and certain disabled individuals. The basic Medicare benefit package (termed "Original Medicare" in this report) provides broad protection against the costs of many, primarily acute, health care services. However, Medicare beneficiaries may still have significant additional costs. Medicare requires beneficiaries to pay part of the cost for most covered services, provides only limited protection for some services (e.g., medical costs incurred outside of the United States), and provides no protection for other services (e.g., custodial long-term care, hearing aids, and dentures). Furthermore, unlike most large group health insurance policies, Original Medicare contains no upper ("catastrophic") limit on out-of-pocket expenses. As a result, Medicare beneficiaries have the potential to incur high out-of-pocket costs for their health care.

Most Medicare beneficiaries therefore have some form of (private or public) additional coverage to supplement some or all of their out-of-pocket costs for Medicare benefits. *Medigap* is one form of private supplemental coverage; Medigap fills some of the cost gaps left by Medicare, such as deductibles, coinsurance, and copayments.[1] In order to be eligible to purchase Medigap, individuals must be

- enrolled in both Part A (Hospital Insurance) and Part B (Supplementary Medical Insurance) of Original Medicare, and
- not enrolled in Medicare Advantage (an HMO-type plan).

Medigap is financed through beneficiary payments to private insurance firms, although retirees may have premiums paid on their behalf by their former employers. There are no government contributions toward Medigap premiums.

This report provides an overview of Medigap. After a review of Medicare coverage, the report covers the ways in which Medicare is supplemented. A discussion of the Medigap plans includes standardized plans, prestandardized plans, older standardized plans available for renewal only, plans in states with Medigap waivers, SELECT plans, and high-deductible plans. The analysis then covers various consumer protections, and the requirements for the insurance companies that offer Medigap. Next, the role of the National Association of Insurance Commissioners (NAIC), a nongovernmental advisory body, is discussed. The report then provides an empirical picture of Medigap markets.

The report concludes with a discussion of two current policy issues. First, how much of the total collected premiums might each insurer be expected to return to its beneficiaries as payment for claims? Second, what is the potential effect on Medicare spending and the federal deficit of increasing the share of health care costs that the individual must pay out of his or her own pocket? Individuals on average reduce their use of medical care following an increase in the price of care. The decrease in medical care by Medicare beneficiaries could lead to a reduction in aggregate

---

[1] Medigap is also known as *Medicare Supplement* Insurance. Cost-sharing refers to the amount paid by the individual for Medicare-allowable goods and services (excluding premiums). Cost-sharing includes a *deductible*, or a set dollar amount the beneficiary must pay before Medicare provides any reimbursement for most services. Cost-sharing also includes *copayments* and/or *coinsurance*, with Medicare paying the remaining (allowable) costs. In general usage, copayment refers to a flat amount (e.g., $30 per visit), whereas coinsurance refers to a percentage (e.g., 20% of the total visit charge).

Medicare expenditures and a reduction in the deficit. On the other hand, the beneficiaries could experience deteriorations in health status if they reduce their use of medical services, which could lead to an ultimate increase in the amount and cost of necessary care, and an increase in Medicare spending and the deficit.

## Medicare Coverage

Medicare consists of four parts:

- Part A, Hospital Insurance (HI), covers inpatient hospital services, skilled nursing care, some home health care, and hospice care.
- Part B, Supplementary Medical Insurance (SMI), covers physician and non-physician practitioner services, outpatient services, some home health, durable medical equipment, clinical laboratory and other diagnostic tests, preventive services, Part B drugs and biologics, and other medical services.
- Part C, Medicare Advantage (MA, a private plan option for beneficiaries), covers all Part A and Part B services, except hospice care.[2]
- Part D covers prescription drug benefit.

Together, Part A and Part B of Medicare comprise Original Medicare, which covers benefits on a fee-for-service (FFS) basis. Currently, most Medicare beneficiaries choose Original Medicare, obtaining covered services through the providers of their choice with Medicare paying its share of the bill for each rendered service. Alternatively, about one-fourth of all beneficiaries choose to enroll in a Medicare Advantage plan.

Most individuals aged 65 and over are automatically eligible for premium-free Part A based on either their own or their spouses' work history.[3] Enrollment in Part B is voluntary and requires a premium. Everyone enrolled in Part A and/or Part B can elect Part D, with premiums varying by the Part D plans.

**Table 1** provides a brief overview of the coverage offered under Medicare Part A and Part B, along with the associated cost-sharing.[4]

---

[2] Most beneficiaries enrolled in Medicare Advantage can only receive prescription drugs through their plan. Only those enrolled in a Medicare Private Fee-for-Service MA plan may purchase a stand-alone Part D prescription drug plan.

[3] Most individuals do not pay a premium for Part A because they or their spouses paid at least 40 quarters of Medicare payroll taxes while working.

[4] Home health services, community health services, some preventive services, and some other services are not subject to the Part B deductible.

### Table 1. Select Original Medicare Cost-Sharing Levels, 2012

| Benefits | Cost-Sharing for Beneficiaries |
|---|---|
| **Medicare Part A** | |
| Inpatient hospital stay, per benefit period | |
|     Days 1-60 | $1,156 deductible |
|     Days 61-90 | $289 per day |
|     Lifetime reserve days (up to 60) | $578 per day |
|     Additional days | 100% |
| Hospice care | |
|     Care | $0 |
|     Prescriptions | Up to $5 |
|     Inpatient respite care | 5% |
| Skilled nursing facility care, per benefit period | |
|     Days 1-20 | $0 |
|     Days 21-100 | $144.50 per day |
|     After day 100 | 100% |
| Part A deductible | (see hospital, Days 1-60, above) |
| **Medicare Part B** | |
| Medical and other services (includes physicians) | 20% |
| Outpatient treatment of mental health services | 40% |
| Excess charges | No coverage of excess charges |
| Part B deductible | $140 |
| **Blood** | 100% of the cost of reimbursement for the actual expense of blood (if any) and for the processing and service charges for the first 3 pints inside and/or outside the hospital; copayment after the first three pints outside the hospital |
| **Foreign travel emergency** | No coverage of foreign travel emergencies |
| **Out-of-pocket limit** | No out of pocked limit |

**Sources:** Centers for Medicare & Medicaid Services, *Medicare and You*, 2012, pp. 31-54 and pp. 59-65, http://www.medicare.gov/publications/pubs/pdf/10050.pdf, and Centers for Medicare & Medicaid Services, *FAQ: Frequently Asked Questions About Medicare*, October 27, 2011, https://questions.medicare.gov/app/answers/detail/a_id/2309/kw/2012%20DEDUCTABLE.

**Notes:** Cost-sharing is waived for certain screenings and preventive services. The deductible is waived for home health services, community health services, preventive services, and some other services. A benefit period begins the day the beneficiary is admitted to a hospital or skilled nursing facility, and ends when the beneficiary has not received hospital or skilled nursing care for 60 consecutive days. Excess charges are the difference between the Medicare approved amount and actual charges, subject to charge limitations set by Medicare or state law. There is a 190-day limit on lifetime inpatient mental health care days.

Medicare does not cover all medical goods and services, including custodial long-term care, routine dental care, dentures, vision care, cosmetic surgery, acupuncture, most care received in other countries, charges above what Medicare reimburses, and hearing aids, among others.[5] There is no out-of-pocket limit under Original Medicare.

Alternatively, some beneficiaries are enrolled in Medicare Advantage (MA), which is also known as Part C. These beneficiaries obtain all covered Medicare services except hospice care through private policies, such as health maintenance organizations (HMOs). Some Part C enrollees may be offered additional benefits beyond what is available in Original Medicare; the scope of additional benefits varies by the health insurance plan. MA plans may include drugs through MA-PD (prescription drug) plans. Individuals who are enrolled in an MA plan may not be sold a Medigap plan.[6]

## Supplementing Medicare

Many individuals have additional health insurance coverage to help pay for some of the costs that Medicare does not cover. **Figure 1** presents the breakdown across supplemental coverage types in 2008.[7]

---

[5] For more information on Medicare, see CRS Report R40425, *Medicare Primer*, coordinated by Patricia A. Davis.

[6] If an individual purchased a Medigap plan prior to enrolling in MA, he or she may continue to enroll in the Medigap plan. The Medigap plan, however, cannot cover deductibles, copayments, coinsurance, or premiums under the MA plan. For more information, see Centers for Medicare & Medicaid Services, *Medicare and You*, 2012, p. 68, http://www.medicare.gov/publications/pubs/pdf/10050.pdf.

[7] This report cites studies that generally use one of two data sources. The first data source is the National Association of Insurance Commissioners (NAIC). The NAIC is an association of insurance regulators from the 50 states, Washington, DC, and four U.S. territories. The NAIC collects financial information from insurance companies. Data collected by the NAIC is administrative data, and provides relatively more detailed information on the characteristics of Medigap plans sold. The second data source is the Access to Care file of the Medicare Current Beneficiary Survey (MCBS), which includes self-reported data on whether an individual holds a Medigap plan. The survey data provides relatively more detailed information on the characteristics of the Medigap plan beneficiaries. These two data sources are not necessarily comparable.

Moreover, estimates from different organizations may not be comparable even when the same data source is used. For example, both the Kaiser Family Foundation and the Office of the Assistant Secretary for Policy Evaluation (ASPE) of the Department of Health and Human Services use data from the Access to Care file of the MCBS, but the organizations' estimates are not comparable. At a minimum, these organizations define variables slightly differently, and differ in their treatment of missing values.

**Figure 1. Sources of Supplemental Coverage Among Medicare Beneficiaries, 2008**

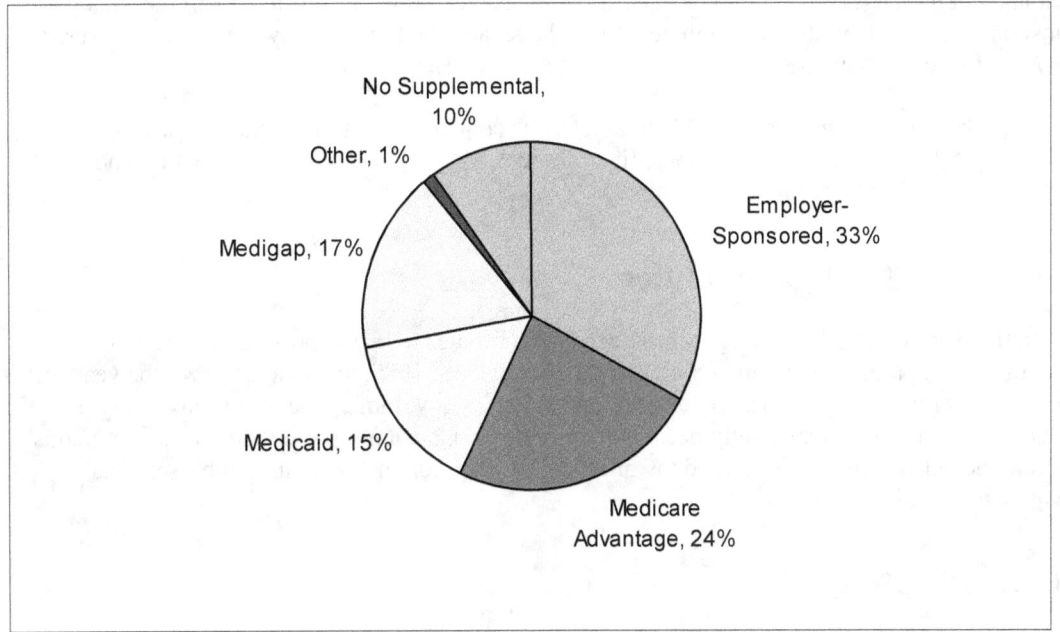

**Source:** Juliette Cubanski, Jennifer Huang, and Anthony Damico, et al., *Medicare Chartbook*, The Henry J. Kaiser Family Foundation, November 2010, p. 60, http://www.kff.org/medicare/upload/8103.pdf.

**Notes:** Data are from the Medicare Current Beneficiary Survey, Access to Care File, 2008. Employer-sponsored insurance includes retiree drug subsidies and TRICARE (the military health care program). All of the pie pieces are mutually exclusive in that once an individual has one type of supplemental insurance (or none), he or she cannot have another type. Supplemental coverage was assigned in the following order: (1) Medicare Advantage, (2) Medicaid, (3) Employer-Sponsored Insurance, (4) Medigap, (5) Other, and (6) No supplemental coverage. Individuals with more than one source of coverage were assigned to the category that appears highest in the ordering.

Only 10% of the Medicare population had no supplemental coverage; these individuals relied solely on Original Medicare. The largest group of individuals (33%) of all Medicare beneficiaries received supplemental coverage from their employers. The next largest group of individuals (24%) were enrolled in Medicare Advantage. Medigap (17%) and Medicaid (15%) were other sources of supplemental insurance.[8]

## Medigap Plans

Medigap policies are sold in both the individual and the group health insurance markets. Whether purchased in the individual or the group market, each Medigap policy covers one individual.[9]

---

[8] *Medicaid* is a means-tested individual entitlement program that finances the delivery of primary care medical services, acute care medical services, and long-term care services and supports. Within broad federal guidelines, each state designs and administers its own program.

[9] A group health policy is defined in Section 5000(a)(1) of the Internal Revenue Code to mean "a plan (including a self-insured plan) of, or contributed to by, an employer (including a self-employed person) or employee organization to provide health care (directly or otherwise) to the employees, former employees, the employer, others associated or formerly associated with the employer in a business relationship, or their families."

Plans are identified by letter, and each plan is associated with a specific benefit package. For example, all Plan As have the same benefit package. The term "plan" refers to all the Medigap insurance contracts with a common benefit package, and the term "policy" refers to an insurance contract sold by an insurer to a beneficiary (e.g., United Healthcare's Plan A).

Federal law governing the sale of Medigap plans is contained in section 1882 of the Social Security Act. This section of the report first provides a history of Medigap legislation and then characterizes the various Medigap plans.

## History of Medigap Statutes

Health insurance regulation largely has been and continues to be the province of the states; Medigap is a partial exception.[10] Medigap reform began in 1980, and changes over the years can be characterized along several dimensions. What began as voluntary standards governing the behavior of insurers increasingly became requirements. Consumer protections were continuously strengthened, and there was a trend toward the simplification of Medigap reimbursements whenever possible.

### During the 1980s

The federal government first provided a *voluntary* certification option for Medigap insurers in Section 507 of the Social Security Disability Amendments of 1980 (P.L. 96-265), commonly known as the "Baucus Amendment." To meet the Baucus Amendment's *voluntary* minimum standards, the Medigap plan was required to

- meet or exceed the NAIC model standards for such plans, and
- return to policyholders as aggregate benefits at least 75% of the aggregate amount of premiums collected in group policies and at least 60% of the aggregate amount collected in individual policies.

Whether or not the insurers met these voluntary standards, the Secretary of Health, Education, and Welfare (now Health and Human Services, HHS) was required to

- make information available to Medicare beneficiaries about the value of Medigap policies,
- study the methods the states used to regulate Medigap plans, and
- report to Congress, at least once every two years, on the effectiveness of the certification procedure.

The move toward increased consumer protections was evident beginning in the late 1980s. The Medicare and Medicaid Patient and Program Protection Act of 1987 (P.L. 100-93) provided that individuals who knowingly and willfully make a false statement or misrepresent a medical fact in the sale of Medigap are guilty of a felony. The Omnibus Budget Reconciliation Act of 1987 (P.L.

---

[10] For information on the federal regulation of pension plans, health plans, and other employee benefit plans, see archived CRS Report RL34443, *Summary of the Employee Retirement Income Security Act (ERISA)*, by Patrick Purcell and Jennifer Staman.

100-203, OBRA87) permitted the participating physicians or suppliers to be paid directly by the Medigap plans.

The Medicare Catastrophic Coverage Act of 1988 (P.L. 100-360, MCCA) improved the information available to potential Medigap purchasers by directing the Secretary of HHS to inform them about sales abuses, publish a toll-free phone number to report such abuses, and inform potential beneficiaries of the addresses and telephone numbers of state and federal offices that provide information and assistance. MCCA also *required* that Medigap plans offered in a state meet or exceed the NAIC guidelines; if this requirement was not met, federal model standards would be established for that state.

Several provisions in MCAA would have made additional changes to Medicare, but they were repealed (before they went into effect) by the Medicare Catastrophic Coverage Repeal Act of 1989 (P.L. 101-234), The changes included

- expanding Medicare Part B benefits,
- imposing an annual supplemental Medicare premium on Part A beneficiaries whose tax liability equaled or exceed $150, and
- imposing an out-of-pocket maximum on Part B expenditures.

These changes would generally have lowered the Medicare beneficiary's level of cost-sharing, and therefore interact with Medigap.

## During the 1990s

The Omnibus Budget Reconciliation Act of 1990 (P.L. 101-508, OBRA90) replaced some voluntary guidelines with federal standards. In particular, OBRA90

- provided for the sale of only 10 standardized Medigap plans (in all but three states);
- guaranteed plan renewability (with rare exceptions);
- prohibited the selling of policies that duplicated certain health insurance provisions to which a beneficiary was entitled, for instance through a retiree health plan;
- curtailed the use of preexisting condition limitations and other forms of health-based pricing;
- required that insurers return to policyholders as aggregate benefits at least 75% of the aggregate amount of premiums collected in group policies and at least 65% of the aggregate amount collected in individual policies; and
- introduced Medigap SELECT plans in 15 states, where SELECT plans provided a managed-care option for beneficiaries with reimbursement within a limited network.

The Act to Amend the Omnibus Budget Reconciliation Act of 1990, which was passed in 1995 (P.L. 104-18), extended the 15-state Medicare SELECT demonstration program to every state, at state option.

Two of the statutes enacted during the 1990s continued to emphasize consumer protections. The Balanced Budget Act of 1997 (P.L. 105-32, BBA97) imposed restrictions on preexisting condition exclusions during the initial Medigap open-enrollment period when the plan purchaser is at least age 65 and meets a requirement for previous health insurance coverage. In addition, the BBA97 requested that the Secretary of HHS ask the NIAC to develop two high-deductible Medigap plans, which became known as Plan F—High Deductible Version and Plan J. The Ticket to Work and Work Incentives Improvement Act of 1999 (P.L. 106-170) permitted disabled Medicare beneficiaries to request the suspension of Medigap when they were covered under a major medical group health policy.

A few Medigap statutes passed in the 1990s primarily affected the insurance firms. The Social Security Act Amendments of 1994 (P.L. 103-432, SSAA94) modified OBRA90. As listed above, OBRA90 barred the sale of policies that duplicated other (non-Medigap) coverage to which a beneficiary was entitled. OBRA90 therefore had the unintended consequence of insurers refusing to sell Medigap policies to beneficiaries who had any other type of private coverage, however limited. SSAA94 amended the OBRA90 requirements by narrowing the anti-duplication provisions and clarifying the circumstances under which insurers could sell health insurance policies with duplicative (non-Medigap) coverage.

The Omnibus Consolidation and Emergency Supplemental Appropriation Act of 1999 (P.L. 105-277) required that providers or facilities that paid Medigap premiums for beneficiaries be subject to civil penalties. This legislation attempted to avoid conflicts of interest created when providers or facilities first paid premiums and then self-referred patients.

## During the 2000s

The Consolidated Appropriations Act, 2001 (P.L. 106-554) specified various anti-discrimination provisions. In particular, individuals who experienced certain changes in their health insurance status (e.g., involuntary termination of a Medigap plan) were guaranteed the right to purchase a new Medigap plan and were protected against preexisting conditions exclusions.

The Medicare Prescription Drug Improvement and Modernization Act of 2003 (P.L. 108-173, MMA) included various changes in Medigap plans. Because the MMA added the Medicare Part D drug provisions, Medigap plans containing drug benefits could no longer be sold to those who did not already have them. Those whose Medigap policies were issued before January 1, 2006, and did contain drug coverage were allowed to keep their existing Medigap policy as is, in some cases to keep their existing policy minus the drug benefit, or to purchase Medicare Part D together with either their old Medigap plan minus the drug benefit or certain new Medigap plans. In particular, individuals with Medigap Plan H, Plan I, and Plan J were guaranteed the right to purchase any of Plan A, Plan B, Plan C, and Plan F with the same insurance carrier. Moreover, the carrier could not use the individual's health status, claims experience, receipt of health care, or medical condition to determine the premium. Excluding preexisting conditions from these policies was also prohibited.

The MMA also requested that the Secretary of HHS request the NAIC to develop additional Medigap plans. Two plans were to incorporate coinsurance and a maximum out-of-pocket limit; no plans available in 2003 had these features. These two plans became Plan K and Plan L. Any other Medigap plans developed by the NAIC did not have to incorporate these features, but were required to exclude prescription drug benefits; Plan M and Plan N fell into this category. In some instances, the MMA changes created two identical plans; existing Medigap Plan E, Plan H, Plan I, and Plan J were eliminated because they duplicated other plans.[11]

The Medicare Improvements for Patients and Providers Act of 2008 (P.L. 110-275, MIPPA) set standards for which plans insurers must offer. In particular, insurers who wanted to offer plans beyond the basic least comprehensive plan (Plan A) were required to offer at least one of the most comprehensive plans (Plan C or Plan F). The Genetic Information Nondiscrimination Act of 2008 (P.L. 110-343, GINA) prohibited discrimination by health insurers and employers based on genetic information. Finally, Section 3210 of the Patient Protection and Affordable Care Act of 2010 (P.L. 111-148, ACA, as amended) requested that the Secretary of HHS request that the NAIC "review and revise" cost-sharing in Plan C and Plan F.

## Coordination of Payment Between Medicare and Medigap

The rules governing coordination of the health insurance payments from the insurers to the Medicare service providers for services covered by Medicare Part B are mandated by Section 1842(h)(3)(B) of the Social Security Act.[12] In most cases, when a beneficiary receives care covered by Medicare Part B, the Medicare contractor pays the provider its portion of the bill. The claim is automatically forwarded to the Medigap insurer, and the Medigap insurer pays the provider its portion of the bill. Some insurers also provide this service for Medicare Part A.[13]

## Plan Characteristics

This section first describes the 10 (current) standardized Medigap plans that differ in their deductibles, copayments, coinsurance, and covered services. The section then describes the nonstandard plans: prestandardized plans, older standardized plans available for renewal only, plans in states with Medigap waivers, SELECT plans, and high-deductible plans. Unless otherwise noted, the text refers to those who qualify for Medicare because they are at least age 65; Medigap options for those who qualify for Medicare because they are under age 65 and disabled are discussed later in the report.

The current standardized plans are the third generation of Medigap plans included in statue. The first group of plans predated the plan standardization mandated by OBRA90. The second group of plans (labeled Plan A through Plan J) were standardized and became effective in a state when the terms of OBRA90 were adopted by the state, which was often in 1992.

### Standardized Plans

**Table 2** provides information on the 10 current, standardized Medigap plans. These plans became effective on June 1, 2010, and an individual purchasing a Medigap policy for the first time (in a state without a waiver) must choose among these plans. However, not every Medigap plan is offered in each state.

---

[11] Centers for Medicare & Medicaid Services, "Medicare Program: Recognition of NAIC Model Standards for Regulation of Medicare Supplemental Insurance," 74 *Federal Register* 18810, April 24, 2009.

[12] No comparable statute exists for Part A.

[13] Centers for Medicare & Medicaid Services, *Choosing a Medigap Policy: A Guide to Health Insurance for People with Medicare*, 2012, p. 20, http://www.medicare.gov/publications/pubs/pdf/02110.pdf.

### Table 2. Standard Medigap Plans, Effective On or After June 1, 2010

| Medigap Benefits | A | B | C | D | F | G | K | L | M | N |
|---|---|---|---|---|---|---|---|---|---|---|
| Medicare Part A coinsurance and hospital costs up to an additional 365 days after Medicare benefits are used up | yes | yes | yes | yes | yes | yes | yes | yes | yes | yes |
| Hospice care coinsurance or copayment | yes | yes | yes | yes | yes | yes | 50% | 75% | yes | yes |
| Skilled nursing facility care coinsurance | | | yes | yes | yes | yes | 50% | 75% | yes | yes |
| Medicare Part A deductible | | yes | yes | yes | yes | yes | 50% | 75% | 50% | yes |
| Medicare Part B Coinsurance or Copayment | yes | yes | yes | yes | yes | yes | 50% | 75% | yes | yes (possible) copay) |
| Medicare Part B excess charge | | | | | yes | yes | | | | |
| Medicare Part B deductible | | | yes | | yes | | | | | |
| Blood | yes | yes | yes | yes | yes | yes | 50% | 75% | yes | yes |
| Foreign travel emergency (up to plan limits) | | | yes | yes | yes | yes | | | yes | yes |
| Out-of-pocket limit in 2012 | | | | | | | $4,660 | $2,330 | | |

**Source:** Centers for Medicare & Medicaid Services, *Choosing a Medigap Policy: A Guide to Health Insurance for People with Medicare*, 2012, p. 11, http://www.medicare.gov/publications/pubs/pdf/02110.pdf and Centers for Medicare & Medicaid Services, *K & L Out-of-Pocket Limits Announcements*, September 2011, https://www.cms.gov/Medigap/04_KandL.asp.

**Notes:** This table lists plans available for purchase by new Medigap enrollees as of June 1, 2010. Some of the plans had different benefits before this time. For example, the pre-June 1, 2010, Plan G contained an 80% Medicare Part B excess charge benefit and an at-home recovery benefit, while the post June 1, 2010, Plan G contained a 100% Medicare Part B excess charge benefit and no at-home recovery benefit. A "yes" in a cell indicates that Medigap covers 100% of the cost of the benefit. A percentage in a cell gives the percentage of the cost that Medigap covers. Plan K and Plan L pay 100% of covered services after the Medigap out-of-pocket limit is met. Plan N pays 100% of the Part B coinsurance, except for a copayment of up to $20 for some office visits and up to $50 for emergency room visits that do not result in an inpatient admission. Plan F is also available with a high-deductable option, where the deductible is $2,070 in 2012. Excess charges are the difference between Medicare's recognized amount and actual charges, subject to charge limitations set by Medicare and state law.

These 10 plans differ with respect to generosity of benefits, cost-sharing provisions, deductibles, and other features. Plan A provides a basic set of benefits, and plan F has the most generous benefits. Plan C and Plan F cover all Medicare copayments and deductibles, and therefore provide "first dollar" or "wraparound" coverage for all covered services.[14]

Plan K and Plan L represent a move away from first dollar coverage. In addition to their outpatient copayments, these plans have "catastrophic coverage," in that once the beneficiary has exceeded an annual out-of-pocket spending limit, Medigap pays 100% of the covered costs for the remainder of the insurance year.

---

[14] First dollar coverage of a good or service means that the insurance plan covers 100% of the cost of the good or service (up to any maximum). All plans have first-dollar coverage for preventive care and certain other services.

Plan N pays 100% of the Part B coinsurance, except for a copayment of up to $20 for some office visits and up to $50 for an emergency room visit that does not result in an inpatient admission.

It should be noted that standardization is not absolute; rather, it serves as a national benefit floor within each plan. In each state, Medigap insurers are permitted, with the prior approval of the state insurance commissioner, to offer plans with new or innovative benefits.[15] For example, a version of Plan F offered by Regence Blue Shield of Idaho offers preventive dental benefits.[16] New or innovative benefits, however, may not be used to reduce standardized benefits.

## Prestandardized Plans

Medigap plans offered before OBRA90 became effective are known as prestandardized plans. Although these plans cannot be sold to new beneficiaries, individuals who already have them may keep them. In other words, prestandardized plans are grandfathered as long as the insurer continues to offer them.

## Older Standardized Plans Available for Renewal Only

Older standardized Medigap plans that were once available for purchase but are now only available for renewal are Plan E, Plan H, Plan I, and Plan J. An individual who purchased one of these plans may continue to renew his or her plan provided the insurer keeps offering the plan.[17] However, the insurer may not sell these plans to new enrollees. As with prestandardized plans, older standardized plans are grandfathered.

There is considerable variation among the benefit packages offered by these older plans. Some benefits no longer offered to new beneficiaries may be covered in these plans. For example, Plan H, Plan I, and Plan J can include drug coverage (as long as the beneficiary is not enrolled in Medicare Part D). Those who did not elect Part D may keep the drug benefits in their Medigap plans.[18] A second example of variation is the at-home recovery benefit, which is currently available in Plan D, Plan G, Plan I, and Plan J if the plans were originally sold before May 31, 2010.[19]

## Medigap Plans for States with Waivers

The standardized Medigap plans do not apply to residents of Massachusetts, Minnesota, and Wisconsin.[20] These states had their own standardized Medigap plans prior to the enactment of the federal standardization requirements. The insurance carriers were permitted to continue existing

---

[15] 74 *Federal Register* 18823.

[16] Regence BlueShield of Idaho, "Regence Bridge Medigap (Medicare Supplement) Plans," p. 8, http://www.regence.com/docs/ID/medicare2011/medigap-sales-brochure.pdf.

[17] Centers for Medicare & Medicaid Services, "Medicare Program: Recognition of NAIC Model Standards for Regulation of Medicare Supplemental Insurance," 74 *Federal Register* 18825, April 24, 2009.

[18] For information on the conditions under which Medigap with drug benefits and Part D could be exchanged, see Center for Medicare & Medicaid Services, *Your Guide to Medicare Prescription Drug Coverage*, revised May 2009, pp. 37-54, http://www.medicare.gov/Publications/Pubs/pdf/11109.pdf.

[19] Medicare Interactive, http://www.medicarerights.org/pdf/Pre-2010Medigap-Benefits-National-2012update.pdf.

[20] 74 *Federal Register* 18809.

state standardized plans. The states, however, were required to modify their regulatory requirements to comply with the MMA requirements (e.g., the prohibition against renewing Medigap policies with prescription drug coverage for those enrolled in Medicare Part D). The Medigap plans themselves are broadly similar to the nationally standardized plans, although they differ in their details. For example, at the time these states were granted waivers, their mandated benefits differed. In addition, Wisconsin now covers 40 visits of home health care in addition to those covered by Medicare.[21]

### SELECT Plans

Medicare SELECT plans are Medigap plans that provide beneficiaries with a managed-care option with reimbursement for medical goods and services received within a limited network. Medicare SELECT is available in some states.[22] Purchasers of SELECT plans are required (except in emergencies) to obtain care through specified hospitals and, in some cases, doctors in order to have the SELECT plans pay for services rendered.[23] The beneficiaries' premiums are generally lower in SELECT plans in exchange for the restrictions in provider choice.

### High-Deductible Plans

A second version of Medigap Plan F has a high deductible.[24] In a high-deductible Plan F, all copayments are paid for after the deductible is met. The premium for this plan should be less expensive than the standard (no-deductible) Plan F because a high-deductible often increases the beneficiary's out-of-pocket expenses, all else equal. The 2012 high deductible is $2,070. In addition, a second version of older Medigap Plan J is a grandfathered high-deductible plan.

## Plan Enrollment

Over one-half of Medigap beneficiaries choose one of two plans. **Figure 2** provides the distribution of Medigap participants across all plans. In 2010, about 44% of beneficiaries purchased Plan F. This plan is the most comprehensive available and covers, in addition to the basic services covered in Plan A, all Medicare deductibles, copayments, and excess charges. An additional 14% of beneficiaries purchased Plan C, which includes the same benefits as Plan F, except it does not cover excess charges. In other words, the two most popular benefit plans cover all deductibles and copayments.

---

[21] Center for Medicare & Medicaid Services, *2012 Choosing a Medigap Policy: A Guide to Health Insurance for People with Medicare*, December 2011, pp. 42-44, http://www.medicare.gov/Publications/Pubs/pdf/02110.pdf, and Center for Medicare & Medicaid Services, *Medicare and Home Health Care*, May 2010, http://www.medicare.gov/publications/pubs/pdf/10969.pdf.

[22] 74 *Federal Register* 18823. The insurance contracts for these *Medigap* plans are known as *Medicare* SELECT.

[23] Medicare always pays its share for services whether or not the provider is a SELECT provider.

[24] 74 *Federal Register* 18809.

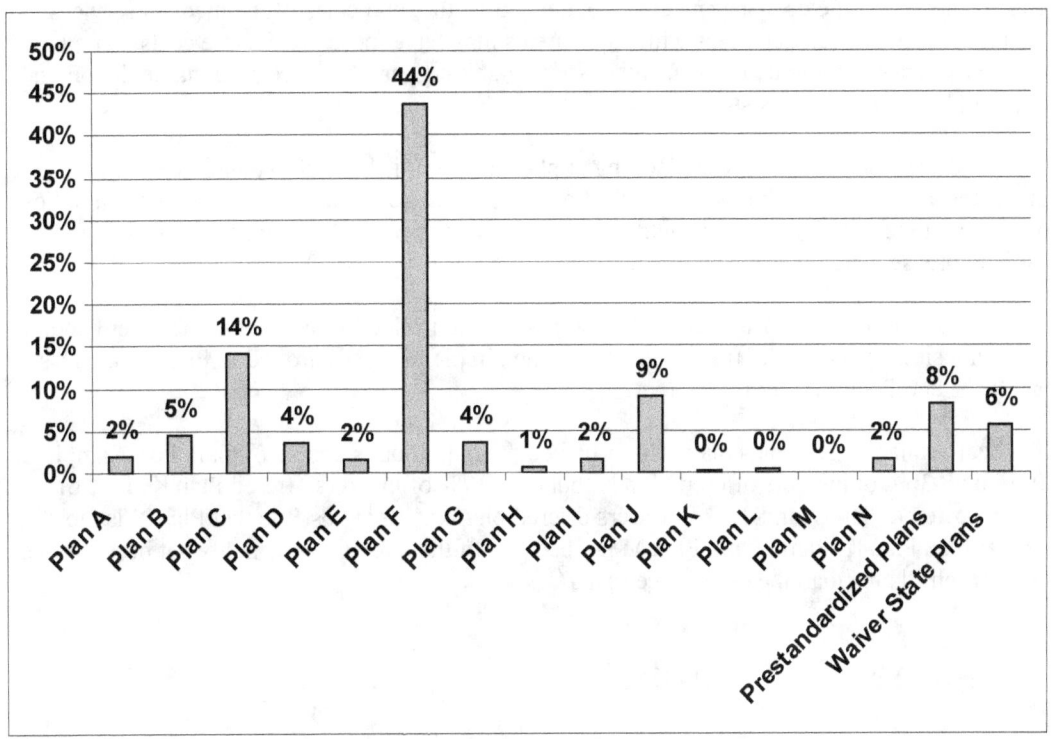

**Figure 2. Distribution of Medigap Plans, All Medigap Beneficiaries, 2010**

**Source:** Assistant Secretary for Planning and Evaluation, U.S. Department of Health and Human Services, *Variation and Trends in Medigap Premiums*, ASPE Report, December 2011, p. 15, http://aspe.hhs.gov/health/reports/2011/MedigapPremiums/index.shtml. The underlying data are from the NAIC.

**Notes:** Note that some of the plans were available for renewal only to long-time policyholders and could not be purchased by other individuals. Totals may not add to 100% because of rounding. Each state with a waiver (Massachusetts, Minnesota, and Wisconsin) offers its own standardized Medigap plans. The waiver state category also contains about 0.6% of the total number of plans that are of unknown type but are primarily issued in Illinois.

Five plans have entered the Medigap market since 2006.[25] Sales of high-deductible Plan F, Plan K, and Plan L began in 2006, and sales of Plan M and Plan N began in 2010. These new plans have different types of cost-sharing.[26] Plan K and Plan L were the first plans to cover less than 100% of the cost of certain benefits including the Medicare Part A deductible and the Part B coinsurance and copayment. Plan K and Plan L cap out-of-pocket spending to compensate for the potentially large costs of these excluded benefits. Plan M covers 50% of the Part A deductible and does not have a cap on out-of-pocket spending. For these three plans, beneficiaries might have a relatively hard time predicting their annual costs because their costs depend on the amount and total cost of the medical services they use. On the other hand, Plan N imposes a $20 copayment for some office visits and up to a $50 copayment for emergency room visits that do not result in an inpatient admission. Under Plan N, beneficiaries might have a relatively easier time predicting

---

[25] The five plans are Plan K and Plan L (whose development by NAIC was requested by the MMA), high-deductible Plan F (which was described in the BBA97), and Plan M and Plan N,

[26] All information in this paragraph is from American's Health Insurance Plans, *Trends in Medigap Coverage and Enrollment, 2011*, May 2012. Information on high-deductible Plan F was collected in a different and less reliable way than information on the other plans.

their annual costs because, while the individual's cost-sharing will vary depending on the number of visits they have, the cost-sharing does not depend on the total costs of the medical services provided. In short, Medigap plans with copayments may have more predictable costs than plans with coinsurance, all else equal. Thus plan N's cost-sharing may be more predictable than Plan K's, Plan L's, or Plan M's cost-sharing.

Because these plans are new, when looking at plan choice, it is helpful to compare their uptake across new enrollees. In other words, the following comparison looks at those choosing a policy for the first time. The individuals could choose between the plans that were available before 2006, and those which became available in 2006.

In 2011, 18% of those choosing a plan for the first time enrolled in Plan N. On the other hand, of those choosing a plan for the first time, 2% enrolled in plan K, 1% enrolled in Plan L, and less than 0.5% enrolled in Plan M.[27]

The local availability of plans may also influence the individual's choice of plan. For example, in 2011 about 36% of insurers offered Plan N, but only 17% of insurers offered Plan K, 15% of insurers offered Plan L, and 8% of insurers offered plan M.[28] It is possible that Plan N is more popular than Plan K, Plan L, and Plan M not because of the known copayments but because more insurers sell Plan N than the other three plans.[29]

# Consumer Protections

This section summarizes the protections accorded to purchasers of Medigap insurance plans who are at least age 65. Consumer protections are strongest during the initial open-enrollment period and are also strong in some circumstances discussed below. The section ends with a discussion of the protections accorded to disabled beneficiaries under age 65.

## During the Open-Enrollment Period

Federal law establishes an initial, one-time six-month Medigap open-enrollment period for the aged that begins on the first day of the first month the individual both is at least 65 and is enrolled in Medicare Part B.[30] Individuals are automatically enrolled in Medicare Part B at age 65.[31]

During the open-enrollment period, the individual is protected in three ways. First, insurers cannot refuse to sell the individual any Medigap policy that the insurer offers. Second, an insurer

---

[27] The high-deductible version of plan F was chosen by between 1% and 3% of new enrollees.

[28] American's Health Insurance Plans, *Trends in Medigap Coverage and Enrollment, 2010-2011*, July 2011, p. 4, http://www.ahipresearch.org/pdfs/Medigap2011.pdf.

[29] If not all insurers offered Plan L or Plan M and if the insurers learned that individuals purchased these plans, when offered, some additional insurers might begin offering them.

[30] 74 *Federal Register* 18825.

[31] Individuals who are covered by employer-sponsored health insurance (ESI), based on either their own on their spouse's active employment, when they turn 65, however, may delay purchasing Part B at that time because they would have to pay a premium for benefits that are (usually) already covered by ESI. The six-month Medigap open-enrollment period for these individuals begins when they purchase Part B, usually when they are no longer covered through ESI based on active employment. Some states have additional open-enrollment periods.

cannot set an individual's policy premiums based on the individual's health (i.e., medical underwriting). Third, insurers cannot impose a waiting period before the individual's policy can start. This third prohibition refers to the start of the entire Medigap policy and is different from a prohibition against the coverage of preexisting conditions.

For the purposes of Medigap, *preexisting conditions* are defined as those conditions diagnosed or treated during the six months immediately preceding the individual's enrollment in a Medigap policy.[32] During open enrollment, individuals may be subject to no more than a six-month preexisting exclusion period. However, preexisting condition limitations may not be imposed at all in certain cases:[33]

- If on the date of application, the individual is in the first six-month enrollment period, and has had at least six months of health insurance coverage meeting the definition of "creditable coverage" under the Health Insurance Portability and Accountability Act of 1996 (P.L. 104-191, HIPAA), he or she cannot have preexisting condition limitations. If the individual has less than six months of creditable coverage, the waiting period for the preexisting conditions is reduced by the number of months of creditable coverage.[34]
- An individual who met the exception for preexisting condition limitations in one Medigap plan does not have to meet the exception under a new plan for previously covered benefits.[35]

## After the Open-Enrollment Period

If an individual applies for a Medigap policy after the open-enrollment period, the insurer is sometimes permitted to use medical underwriting. *Medical underwriting* is the use of an individual's health history to decide whether to accept the health insurance application, whether to add a waiting period for preexisting conditions (if permitted by state law), and how much to charge the individual for his or her Medigap policy.

### Guaranteed Issue

Even after the open-enrollment period has passed, however, the individual may have other consumer protections when purchasing a Medigap policy in limited situations. Medigap *guaranteed issue* rights are the rights to buy a Medigap plan, have all preexisting conditions covered, and not be charged more for past or present health conditions.[36] There are four broad classes of guaranteed issue rights: rights following a change in residence or employment, rights associated with sampling a Medicare Advantage or Medicare SELECT plan (trial rights), rights triggered by certain actions by the insurer (no fault rights), and other rights.

---

[32] 74 *Federal Register* 18818.

[33] Broad limits on the use by insurers of preexisting conditions were imposed by the Health Insurance Portability and Accountability Act of 1996 (P.L. 104-191, HIPAA).

[34] The insurer may impose a preexisting exclusion limitation if the individual did not have such creditable coverage. Creditable coverage generally requires that there has not been a break in health insurance coverage for more than 63 days.

[35] An insurer could impose exclusions for newly covered benefits.

[36] 74 *Federal Register* 18825-18826.

## Rights After Changes in Residence or Employment

If the individual is covered by Medicare, and his or her place of residence or labor force status changes, the individual may have guaranteed issue rights for Plan A, Plan B, Plan C, Plan F, Plan K, and Plan L. In general, to preserve these rights, the individual must apply for the Medigap plan no later than 63 calendar days after the previous health insurance coverage ends. The rights are available for the following reasons:

- An individual is enrolled in a Medicare Advantage plan and moves out of the geographic area. The individual must switch to Original Medicare before the Medigap purchase.

- An individual has Original Medicare and
    - an employer group health policy (including retiree or COBRA coverage), or
    - union coverage that is a secondary payer to Medicare, and the individual's policy ends. If the individual has COBRA coverage, guaranteed issue extends to the end of COBRA.[37] The individual may have additional rights under state law.

- An individual has Medicare SELECT and moves out of the SELECT plan's service area.

## Trial Rights

Some individuals enrolled in Original Medicare may want to try out different Medicare alternatives such as Medicare Advantage or Medicare SELECT. These individuals may switch from Original Medicare to MA or Medicare SELECT, and can try out that policy for up to one year. If these individuals decide to switch back to Original Medicare within that initial year, they are guaranteed the right to enroll in a Medigap policy at that time. These rights operate as follows:

- If the individual joined MA when he or she was first eligible for Medicare Part A at age 65, within the first year of joining, the individual may switch to Original Medicare and have guaranteed issue rights for any standardized Medigap plan sold in the state.[38]

- If the individual dropped a Medigap policy to join an MA or Medicare SELECT plan for the first time, and the individual has been in the new plan for less than a year, the individual has guaranteed issue rights for the original Medigap plan if the former insurer still sells it. If the former plan is not available, the individual

---

[37] COBRA coverage takes its name from the Consolidated Omnibus Budget Reconciliation Act of 1985 (P.L. 99-272). COBRA requires employers with 20 or more employees to provide employees and their families the right to continue participation in the employer's group health policy in case of certain events, one of which is involuntary dismissal. For more information on COBRA, see CRS Report R40142, *Health Insurance Continuation Coverage Under COBRA*, by Janet Kinzer.

[38] The guaranteed issue right also holds if the individual joins the Programs of All-Inclusive Care For the Elderly (PACE). PACE is a capitated benefit permanently authorized by the BBA97 with a comprehensive service delivery system and integrated Medicare and Medicaid financing.

has guaranteed issue rights for any of Medigap Plan A, Plan B, Plan C, Plan F, Plan K, or Plan L that is sold in the state.

These rights generally last for 63 days after coverage of the forfeited MA or SELECT plan ends, although they might last for an extra 12 months under certain circumstances.

### *No Fault Rights*

If an insurer is no longer able to sell the Medigap plan, or has not followed the requirements for Medigap insurers, or has misled the individual, the individual's purchase of Medigap Plan A, Plan B, Plan C, Plan F, Plan K, or Plan L from any insurance carrier is guaranteed as follows:[39]

- If the individual's insurer goes bankrupt or a Medigap policy ends through no fault of the individual, the individual has guaranteed issue rights.
- If the Medigap insurer commits fraud, and the individual then drops the insurer's business, the individual has guaranteed issue rights.

### *Other Rights*

If the individual is enrolled in an MA plan and the insurer sponsoring the plan stops participating in Medicare or if the MA plan leaves the geographic area, the individual has guaranteed issue rights to purchase any of Medigap Plan A, Plan B, Plan C, Plan F, Plan K, and Plan L that is sold in the state by any insurance carrier. The individual must be enrolled in Original Medicare before purchasing Medigap.

### Guaranteed Renewal

Standardized Medigap policies are guaranteed renewable so long as the plan remains for sale in the market.[40] A Medigap insurer may only terminate a beneficiary's standardized plan if that beneficiary commits fraud, makes an untrue statement, or fails to pay the premium.

## Genetic Nondiscrimination

Section 104 of the Genetic Information Nondiscrimination Act (P.L. 110-343, GINA) prohibits Medigap insurers from[41]

- using genetic information about an individual to deny coverage, adjust premiums, or impose preexisting condition exclusions;
- requiring or requesting genetic testing; and
- requesting, requiring, or purchasing genetic information for underwriting purposes.

---

[39] 74 *Federal Register* 18826.

[40] 74 *Federal Register* 18818.

[41] For additional information on GINA, see CRS Report RL34584, *The Genetic Information Nondiscrimination Act of 2008 (GINA)*, by Amanda K. Sarata and James V. DeBergh.

## Switching Medigap Plans

A beneficiary might want to switch Medigap plans to reduce or increase the benefit levels, change the insurance firm, or move to a less expensive plan. To purchase a new Medigap plan, the beneficiary must notify the first Medigap insurer that he or she is going to cancel that insurer's plan as of a certain date. If the new Medigap plan starts one month before the coverage from the old Medigap plan ends, the beneficiary has 30 days to decide whether to keep the new Medigap plan. The beneficiary must pay premiums for both the old and new Medigap plans during these thirty days.[42]

Even though a beneficiary may be able to switch Medigap plans, he or she might not want to. In particular, the consumer rights discussed above do not apply outside of the circumstances listed above. At other times, the insurer might refuse to sell the individual a policy or increase the premium if the individual is in poor health.

## Medigap for Individuals Under Age 65

To be covered under Medicare before age 65, individuals must qualify for Medicare based on disability. In particular, individuals under age 65 who received cash disability benefits from Social Security or the Railroad Retirement systems for at least 24 months are entitled to Medicare Part A.[43] While there is no federal requirement that insurers sell Medigap plans to disabled individuals, some states require that Medigap plans be available to some or all of these individuals.[44] In other states, insurers choose to sell Medigap plans even though there is no requirement that they do so. If permitted by state law, insurers can use medical underwriting and charge higher premiums for the standardized plans when selling to those under age 65.

Those under age 65 covered by Medigap are entitled to all open-enrollment rights upon turning 65. Because medical underwriting is forbidden during the initial open-enrollment period, the beneficiary's premium might drop at age 65 because the beneficiary's health status can no longer affect the premium. In addition, for those who have had Medicare for at least six months immediately before turning 65, there is no preexisting condition waiting period because the beneficiaries have met the creditable coverage requirement.

# Insurers' Requirements

In addition to fulfilling these consumer protection requirements, insurers must offer certain plans, set premiums for their Medigap plans, and ensure the plans return a certain amount of the dollar value of claims as benefits to the policy holders.

---

[42] Centers for Medicare & Medicaid Services, *Choosing a Medigap Policy: A Guide to Health Insurance for People with Medicare*, 2012, pp. 32-35, http://www.medicare.gov/publications/pubs/pdf/02110.pdf.

[43] Centers for Medicare & Medicaid Services, *Choosing a Medigap Policy: A Guide to Health Insurance for People with Medicare*, 2011, p. 39-40, http://www.medicare.gov/publications/pubs/pdf/02110.pdf. Many disabilities qualify. In addition, a few specific illnesses/diseases have special provisions for Medicare enrollment; examples include End-Stage Renal Disease (ESRD, or permanent kidney failure requiring dialysis or a kidney transplant) and Amyotrophic Lateral Sclerosis (ALS, also known as Lou Gehrig's disease).

[44] 74 *Federal Register* 18829.

## Required Plans

If an insurer wishes to offer any Medigap plans, the insurer must offer the basic plan (i.e., Plan A). If the insurer wishes to offer any plan(s) in addition to Plan A, the insurer must then offer at least Plan C or Plan F, before it can offer any other plan.[45]

## Premiums

A *rating option* is the method by which the insurer sets premiums for health insurance policies. There are three rating options in the Medigap market. Premiums may increase over time under all three ratings options; the options differ in the conditions under which premiums may increase based on the ratings option. For example, all options allow premiums to vary with the inflation rate in the beneficiary's community, but not all options allow premiums to vary with the beneficiary's age. Depending on the state, premiums may also vary with gender, smoking status, and perhaps other variables. The three rating options are as follows:

- Under the *community rating* option, the premium does not depend on the beneficiary's age. Therefore all individuals enrolled in a particular plan pay the same premium, and it does not increase with the individual's age.

- Under the *issue-age rating* option, the premium is based on the beneficiary's age when the Medigap policy was first purchased. For example, if Plan A is sold by an insurer in Maryland for 2012, that insurer would charge a lower premium for a 65-year-old new enrollee than for a 75-year-old enrollee. However, for any given individual, the premium may not increase as the individual grows older. Premiums are therefore relatively high (when compared to premiums that are adjusted each plan year for an individual's attained age) at the time of initial purchase, but do not increase as the beneficiary ages.

- Under the *attained-age rating* option, the premium is based on the beneficiary's current (attained) age. Premiums are relatively low when the individual first purchases the policy (i.e., those who are 65), but as the individual ages, the premiums will increase.

The greatest difference between the ratings options, therefore, is the way premiums increase (or do not increase) over time. From a beneficiary's perspective, the least expensive option for any given policy at the date of purchase may not be the least expensive option over the lifetime of the policy. When comparing premiums across insurance companies, therefore, individuals need to consider the premiums (or expected premiums) over the lifetime of the policy.

---

[45] 74 *Federal Register* 18823. See also Centers for Medicare & Medicaid Services, *Choosing a Medigap Policy: A Guide to Health Insurance for People with Medicare*, 2012, p. 12, http://www.medicare.gov/publications/pubs/pdf/02110.pdf.

# Medical Loss Ratios

## Definition and Rationale

The *medical loss ratio* (MLR) measures the extent to which an insurance company uses the premiums it receives to cover the claims of its beneficiaries. More precisely, the MLR is the percentage of the total premiums received that the insurance company spends on health care benefits. Thus, if a plan received $100 in premiums and spent $85 on medical claims, its MLR would be 85%. A relatively high MLR suggests that the policy holders are receiving value because they are receiving relatively more benefits, and the insurance company is retaining relatively less in administrative costs and profits. The required Medigap medical loss ratios are at least 75% for group plans and at least 65% for individual plans.[46] Should a Medigap insurer fail to meet the required ratios, the insurer is required to reimburse the beneficiaries by offering refunds or credits in order to meet the Medigap plan MLR requirement.

The required MLR is lower for individual policies than for group policies because an insurance firm's administrative costs tend to be higher for individual plans. For example, it is more expensive (per beneficiary) to market plans to individuals one at a time than it is to market to one employer (or one union or one retiree group) on behalf of multiple individuals.

## Required Calculations

The actual process by which individual insurers calculate their respective MLRs involves more details and assumptions.[47] First, the insurer must calculate the MLR over the lifetime of each Medigap insurance plan (e.g., Plan A, Plan B). By assumption, the lifetime of each Medigap plan is 15 years. Second, each Medigap policy is assumed to pay out a smaller amount of premiums at the start of the policy, when the beneficiary is relatively young. Third, the insurer must have sold enough policies for the MLR calculations to be considered credible.

To illustrate the way in which the insurer calculates MLRs, consider an insurer in the individual Medigap market; this insurer must demonstrate an MLR of 65% for each plan (e.g., Plan A, Plan B). The required annual MLR, however, incorporates the anticipated changes in claims paid out over time using a benchmark. A benchmark is a standard against which the insurer's claims are assessed. The MLR for each year of the policy is compared to a benchmark loss ratio (i.e., a target value given in the *Federal Register* for that plan year).[48] In particular, each insurer first calculates the MLR (for each plan) for the policies in their first year. The MLR for these first-year plans should be at least 40%, the first year benchmark. The MLR for plans in their second year should be at least 55%, and the MLR for plans in their third year should be at least 65%. The benchmark loss ratios continue to increase until reaching 77% in the 12$^{th}$ year, and then stay at that level for the remainder of the 15-year period. These increasing annual MLRs will result in a cumulative medical loss-ratio of at least 65%. An insurer who has met these annual benchmarks

---

[46] In this context, policies issued as a result of the solicitation of individuals through mail or by mass media advertising are considered individual policies.

[47] U.S. General Accounting Office (now called the Government Accountability Office), *Medigap Insurance: Compliance With Federal Standards Has Increased*, HEHS-98-66, March 1998, http://www.gao.gov/archive/1998/he98066.pdf.

[48] 74 *Federal Register* 18872-18875.

for a plan has satisfied the MLR criteria for that plan. To be in compliance with the statute, the insurer needs to meet the MLR for all the plans it offers.

In addition, insurers are permitted to apply a credibility adjustment to the MLR calculation. If there are not a sufficiently large number of policies written, the estimates and calculations are assumed to have less credibility, and the calculated MLR is permitted to be lower before the insurer is required to offer refunds or credits. In the extreme, a policy loss ratio based on less than 500 life-years since its inception is considered not credible, because there are not enough life-years observed to evaluate the actions of the insurer. In this case, no refund or credit by the insurer is required. The MLR in the group market is calculated the same way, but the loss ratio benchmarks are higher in each year because the statutory MLR is 75% and not 65%.[49]

## The Role of the National Association of Insurance Commissioners

The National Association of Insurance Commissioners (NAIC) is an association of insurance regulators from the 50 states, Washington, DC, and four U.S. territories.[50] One of the Association's stated goals is to make state regulation more consistent and uniform.[51] The NAIC also collects financial information from insurance companies; some of the data presented in this report were collected by the NAIC.[52]

The specific provisions (e.g., levels of cost-sharing and types of coverage) of all Medigap plans (excluding those in waiver states) are formulated by the NAIC. Once finalized, the standardized plans are known as *NAIC model standards* for Medigap plans. The NAIC, however, has no authority to monitor whether the states comply with its model standards. Instead, states retain regulatory authority. States must either

- adopt the NAIC model standards and any subsequent revisions, or
- enact regulatory provisions that are more stringent that those in the NAIC model standards or in the regulatory requirements.[53]

If a states fails to adopt the NAIC model standards, the state will be considered out of compliance with federal requirements and will not be permitted to regulate its Medigap market.[54] In this case, the Centers for Medicare & Medicaid Services of HHS would regulate the sale of Medigap plans.

---

[49] 74 *Federal Register* 18829. The MLR statutes are found at SSA, Section 1882(r).

[50] More formally, the NAIC is a private Internal Revenue Code section 501(c)(3) nonprofit association. The NAIC members are the elected or appointed state government officials who, along with their departments and staff, regulate the conduct of insurance companies and agents in their respective state or territory.

[51] For additional goals, see *About the NAIC*, NAIC, http://www.naic.org/index_about.htm.

[52] In some states, not all insurers report to the state insurance commissions and therefore not all insurers report to the NAIC. For example, health insurance issuers regulated by California's Department of Managed Health Care are not required by state regulators to submit data to the NAIC.

[53] 74 *Federal Register* 18809.

[54] Implementation Materials for Revisions to Medigap Model, NAIC, http://www.naic.org/documents/committees_b_senior_issues_medigap_impl_guide.pdf, p.1.

The NAIC has been actively involved in the evolution of the standardized Medigap plans. Changes are made over time to reflect changing health care statutes and practices. For example, a Medigap "preventive care" benefit was eliminated in 2010 because expanded Medicare Part B benefits made the Medigap preventive care benefit unnecessary. More recently, Section 3210 of ACA requests that the Secretary of HHS ask the NAIC to "review and revise" cost-sharing in two Medigap plans.

# Descriptions of Medigap Markets

This section discusses Medigap premiums, the number of insurance firms in each Medigap market (known as market concentration), the level of participation in Medigap across states, and the socio-demographic characteristics of the Medigap beneficiaries. Because Medigap is sold and regulated by states, each state is its own Medigap market.

## Medigap Premiums and Plan Choice

Medigap premiums for the same exact standardized plan (e.g., Plan F) may not be the same across any or all insurers offering that plan in a state. In fact, there is wide variation in Medigap premiums for each plan nationwide. For example, according to one study, the average monthly premium for Medigap Plan F in 2010 was $193 in Maryland, $149 in Virginia, and $170 in Washington, DC.[55]

This variation reflects the geographic variations in the price levels, state regulations, smoking, gender, and possibly other discounts, and the rating structure used. Even controlling for these differences, however, variations in premiums remain.[56] Individuals do not always purchase the least expensive version of their chosen plan. There are a number of hypotheses concerning this behavior:[57]

- Many of the price comparisons are available on the Internet (at the state insurance websites), and some of the elderly are not Internet-savvy.

- There may be cognitive impairment in this age group, and the large number of choices associated with selecting a Medigap plan could prove daunting.

- Potential Medigap beneficiaries may prefer to remain with their existing (pre-Medicare) insurance agent, even though the existing agent may not sell what would be the best plans for these beneficiaries.

- Certain insurers attract individuals through name recognition.[58]

---

[55] Gretchen Jacobson, Tricia Neuman, and Thomas Rice, et al., *Medigap Reform: Setting the Context*, Kaiser Family Foundation, Issue Brief, September 2011, p. 7, http://www.kff.org/medicare/upload/8235-2.pdf.

[56] Nicole Maestas, Mathis Schroeder, and Dana Goldman, *Price Variation in Markets with Homogeneous Goods: The Case of Medigap*, NBER, Working Paper 14679, January 2009, pp. 1-6, http://www.nber.org/papers/w14679.

[57] Ibid.

[58] For example, most individuals have heard of the Blue Cross/Blue Shield insurers. In addition, many individual policies are purchased in conjunction with the AARP. Individuals who contact the AARP about Medigap are referred to United Healthcare and may then go on to purchase individual Medigap policies from this insurance firm. The AARP markets the plans while United Healthcare is the insurer who bears the risk associated with that insurance. At the (continued...)

## Medigap Market Participation by Individuals Across States

**Figure 3** provides the number of Medigap enrollees in 2010 by state. Enrollment varies from a low of 4,221 individuals in Hawaii to a high of 643,156 individuals in Florida. Other states with a high Medigap enrollment include Texas, Pennsylvania, and Illinois. **Figure 3** is informative from a financial perspective in that it indicates which states have relatively more dollars in the Medigap market. However, the map does not provide any information about whether Ohio has a higher Medigap enrollment than North Dakota because a larger number of those eligible for Medigap actually enroll, or simply because Ohio has more residents than North Dakota.

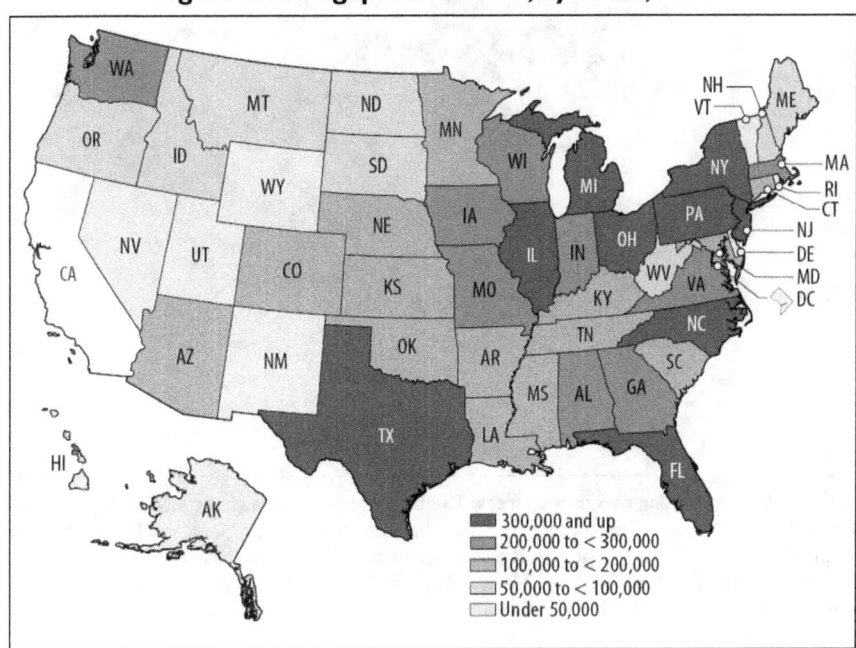

**Figure 3. Medigap Enrollment, by State, 2010**

**Source:** Created by CRS, based on the NAIC data contained in America's Health Insurance Plans, *Trends in Medigap Coverage and Enrollment, 2010-2011*, July 2011, pp. A1-A3, http://www.ahipresearch.org/pdfs/Medigap2011.pdf.

**Notes:** Complete data for California are not available. California has both a Department of Insurance and a Department of Managed Care. These two departments are governed by different regulations, and only the former is required to file data with the NAIC. More information on the Department of Insurance is available at http://insurance.ca.gov. More information on the Department of Managed Care is available at http://www.dmhc.ca.gov.

**Figure 4** shows the percentage of those enrolled in Medicare who purchase Medigap plans, and presents a different picture than **Figure 3**. The percentage of those enrolled in Medicare who purchase Medigap plans is relatively high in parts of the Midwest and mountain states and relatively low in the Southwest. That Medigap policies are popular in the Midwest is consistent

---

(...continued)

national level, United had a national market share of about 46% between 2004 and 2008; see Amanda Starc, *Insurer Pricing and Consumer Welfare: Evidence from Medigap*, Harvard Business School, Working Paper, November 29, 2010, pp 5-9 for details..

with the Medicare Advantage data. In 2011, the participation rate in Medicare Advantage was lower in the Midwest and mountain states than in many other areas of the country.[59] In short, participation is Medicare Advantage is relatively lower in those states where participation in Medigap is relatively high.

**Figure 4. Percent of Medicare Enrollees with Medigap Coverage, by State, 2010**

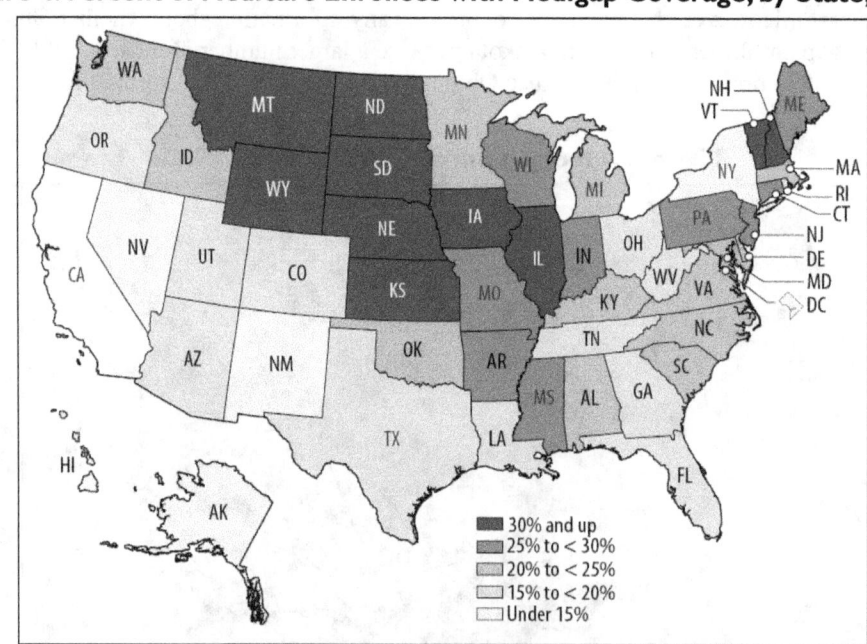

**Source:** CRS calculations using two data sources. The total Medicare data cover July 2010 and are from Table 2.8 of the Medicare & Medicaid Statistical Supplement, https://www.cms.gov/MedicareMedicaidStatSupp/08_2011.asp#TopOfPage. The Medigap data cover December 2010, and are based on NAIC data contained in America's Health Insurance Plans, *Trends in Medigap Coverage and Enrollment, 2010-2011*, July 2011, pp. A1-A3, http://www.ahipresearch.org/pdfs/Medigap2011.pdf.

**Note:** Complete data for California are not available. California has both a Department of Insurance and a Department of Managed Care. These two departments are governed by different regulations, and only the former is required to file data with the NAIC. More information on the Department of Insurance is available at http://insurance.ca.gov. More information on the Department of Managed Care is available at http://www.dmhc.ca.gov.

## Medigap Markets by Characteristics of Enrollees

Limited public information is available on the socio-economic characteristics of those individuals who participate in Medigap. The information reported here comes from various components and years of the Medicare Current Beneficiary Survey. In broad terms, the conclusions across the three studies discussed below are consistent.

A report by America's Health Insurance Plans (AHIP, a trade group) emphasized the differences in take-up rates and socio-economic characteristics between rural and urban beneficiaries in

---

[59] The Henry J. Kaiser Family Foundation, *Medicare: Medicare Advantage*, Fact Sheet, November 2011, p. 1, http://www.kff.org/medicare/upload/2052-15.pdf.

2010.[60] AHIP concluded that 31% of Medigap beneficiaries lived in rural areas, while only 24% of all Medicare beneficiaries did so. AHIP also observed Medigap holders in rural areas were more likely to have lower incomes than their urban peers.

Comprehensive 2007 data are found in the chart pack published by The Henry J. Kaiser Family Foundation.[61] An evaluation of socio-economic characteristics showed that, of those with incomes of $10,000 or less, 7% were covered by Medigap, 7% were covered by employer-sponsored insurance, and 51% were covered by Medicaid. Of those in (self-reported) poor health, 11% were covered by Medigap, but of those in excellent or very good health, 24% were covered by Medigap. Individuals with cognitive impairments were more likely to be covered by Medicaid, and less likely to be covered by either Medigap or employer-sponsored insurance.

Finally, the Medicare Payment Advisory Commission (MedPAC) reported broadly similar results for 2007. Of poor individuals, 13% were covered by Medigap, 9% were covered by employer-sponsored insurance, and 46% were covered by Medicaid. Of those in poor health, 17% were covered by Medigap, but of those in excellent or very good health, 28% were covered by Medigap.[62]

# Current Policy Issues

The focus of current policy issues has been on proposed changes to the Medigap MLR and cost-sharing levels. Background information on these topics was provided above, and current issues are discussed below.

## Increasing Medical Loss Ratios

Companion bills introduced in the 112th Congress, H.R. 2645 and S. 1416, the Medigap Medical Loss Ratio Improvement Act of 2011, seek to increase the medical loss ratio required of Medigap insurers. Currently, comprehensive and major medical health insurance policies (not Medigap policies) sold in the large group market are required to have an 85% MLR, and those sold in the small group and individual markets are required to have an 80% MLR. Insurers who fail to meet these standards must provide rebates to their customers.[63]

Medigap plans have a 75% MLR requirement for the group market and a 65% MLR requirement for the individual market. In other words, private major medical and comprehensive insurers must

---

[60] America's Health Insurance Plans, *Low-Income & Rural Beneficiaries with Medigap Coverage, 2010*, May 2012, http://www.ahipresearch.org/MedigapLowIncomeRuralReport2012.pdf. The underlying data come from the Medicare Current Beneficiary Survey.

[61] Juliette Cubanski, Tricia Neuman, and Anthony Damico, et al., Examining Sources of Supplemental Insurance and Prescription Drug Coverage Among Medicare Beneficiaries: Findings from the Medicare Current Beneficiary Survey, 2007, The Henry J. Kaiser Family Foundation, August 2009, pp. 2-3, http://www.kff.org/medicare/upload/7801-02.pdf. Individuals with employer-sponsored coverage were categorized as employer-sponsored, even if the individuals also carried Medigap.

[62] MedPAC, *Healthcare Spending and the Medicare Program*, June 2011, p. 54, http://www.medpac.gov/documents/Jun11DataBookEntireReport.pdf.

[63] CRS Report R41439, *Health Insurance Agents and Brokers in the Reformed Health Insurance Market*, by Bernadette Fernandez.

return more of the premiums received to their beneficiaries than Medigap insurers must return to their beneficiaries. AARP and others have lobbied for an increase in the Medigap MLRs to the levels found in the comprehensive and major medical health insurance market.[64]

Those in favor of increasing MLRs argue that Medigap enrollees should have the same protections as enrollees of other private health insurance policies. In other words, a low MLR suggests that insurers keep more of claim dollars instead of returning them as benefits. Those opposed to the change argue that Medigap plans have lower premium bases over which to spread administrative costs, and therefore should be allowed to retain greater a share of premiums.[65]

## Increasing Cost-Sharing

Section 3210 of the ACA requires the Secretary of HHS to request the NAIC to "review and revise" the Medigap benefit packages in order to encourage nominal cost-sharing under Plan C and Plan F. Similarly, President Obama's FY2013 budget proposal would provide incentives to increase cost-sharing. Beginning in 2017, the proposal would impose a Part B premium surcharge for new Medicare beneficiaries who select a Medigap plan with low cost-sharing requirements (i.e., offer "near first-dollar" coverage). The surcharge would be equal to approximately 15% of the average Medigap premium. This is equivalent to about 30% of the Part B premium. Moreover, the June 2012 MedPAC Report to the Congress also recommends a new charge for Medigap policies as part of a series of Medicare reforms.[66]

Cost-sharing, by requiring the beneficiary to pay more for some medical care, is often thought to discourage the beneficiary's demand for excessive health services.[67] If this is true, an increase in Medigap cost-sharing might lead to a decrease in medical goods and services used by the beneficiary, and therefore a decrease in Medicare expenditures and the federal deficit.

Some early evidence that an increase in cost-sharing leads to decrease in expenditures was provided by the RAND Health Insurance Experiment (HIE).[68] The HIE randomly assigned individuals under age 65 to "treatments" of various levels of cost-sharing. The HIE evaluation concluded that for every 10% the cost of medical services to the family increased, the family's use of medical services would fall by 2%.

The population of special interest for Medigap is largely individuals aged 65 and over who would experience an increase in cost-sharing for the health insurance policy. These individuals may respond differently than younger adults to changes in cost-sharing for a variety of reasons, including lower and/or fixed incomes, lower levels of health, and uncertainty about their lifespan. Nevertheless, the RAND result has also held up among samples of older individuals, even though

---

[64] Dena Bunis, "Democrats Want New MLR Standards to Apply To Medigap Policies," *CQ Healthbeat News*, July 26, 2011, http://www.cq.com/doc/hbnews-3916554?wr=RDlYTlRja3lSajV1TVYqOXdwRDVWdw. AARP is usually seen as an advocate for senior citizens.

[65] Ibid.

[66] MedPAC, *Medicare and the Health Care Delivery System*, Report to the Congress, June 2012, p. 4, http://www.medpac.gov/documents/jun11_entirereport.pdf,

[67] Willard G. Manning, Joseph P. Newhouse, and Naihua Duan, et al., "Health Insurance and the Demand for Medical Care: Evidence from a Randomized Experiment," *American Economic Review*, vol. 77, no. 3 (June 1987), pp. 251-277.

[68] Willard G. Manning, Joseph P. Newhouse, and Naihua Duan, et al., "Health Insurance and the Demand for Medical Care: Evidence from a Randomized Experiment," *American Economic Review*, vol. 77, no. 3 (June 1987), pp. 251-277.

the RAND experiment did not include individuals over age 64 and was conducted about 30 years ago.[69]

Two additional recent studies conclude that increased financial responsibility reduces medical care use among the elderly, but also illustrate some of the dangers of oversimplifying this matter. One study compared individuals across a staggered set of copayment changes faced by those receiving supplemental health insurance from the California Public Employees Retirement system. The researchers estimated physician visits and prescription drug utilization were "modestly price sensitive" among the elderly.[70] The second study looked at the effects of increased copayments on ambulatory care over time. When their copayments doubled, elderly individuals, when compared with a control group, had almost 20 fewer annual outpatient visits per 100 individuals.[71] However, the cost-sharing issue is more complicated than the above discussion suggests. In the first study, as the individuals reduced their physician visits and prescription drug utilization, the most ill individuals also increased their hospital utilization.[72] In the second study, individuals with increased copayments were sometimes found to have worse health outcomes and an increased total spending on health care.[73] A more complete picture of cost-sharing therefore suggests that increasing copayments can reduce health status among certain populations and ultimately increase health care spending among these populations.[74]

## Author Contact Information

Carol Rapaport
Analyst in Health Care Financing
crapaport@crs.loc.gov, 7-7329

---

[69] Katherine Baicker and Dana Goldman, "Patient Cost-Sharing and Healthcare Spending Growth," *Journal of Economic Perspectives*, vol. 25, no. 2 (Spring 2011), p. 55.

[70] Amitabh Chandra, Jonathan Gruber, and Robin McKnight, "Patient Cost-Sharing and Hospitalization Offsets in the Elderly," *American Economic Review*, vol. 100, no. 1 (March 2010), p. 194.

[71] Amal N. Trivedi, Husein Moloo, and Vincent Mor, "Increased Ambulatory Care Copayments and Hospitalizations among the Elderly," *The New England Journal of Medicine*, vol. 362, no. 4 (January 28, 2010), p. 320.

[72] Amitabh Chandra, Jonathan Gruber, and Robin McKnight, "Patient Cost-Sharing and Hospitalization Offsets in the Elderly," *American Economic Review*, vol. 100, no. 1 (March 2010), p. 194.

[73] Amal N. Trivedi, Husein Moloo, and Vincent Mor, "Increased Ambulatory Care Copayments and Hospitalizations among the Elderly," *The New England Journal of Medicine*, vol. 362, no. 4 (January 28, 2010), p. 320.

[74] Katherine Swartz, *Cost-Sharing: Effects on Spending and Outcomes*, Robert Wood Johnson Foundation, Research Synthesis Report No. 20, December 2010, pp. 1-5, http://www.rwjf.org/files/research/121710.policysynthesis.costsharing.rpt.pdf, and Robert Wood Johnson Foundation, *Cost-Sharing: Effects on Spending and Outcomes*, Policy Brief, December 2010, p. 1, http://www.rwjf.org/files/research/121710.policysynthesis.costsharing.brief.pdf.

www.ingramcontent.com/pod-product-compliance
Lightning Source LLC
Chambersburg PA
CBHW081245180526
45171CB00005B/554